Bedtime Stories for Stressed Out Adults

Deep sleep relaxing stories and meditation to help you heal your body from anxiety and stress

by Martha Peterson

Table of Contents

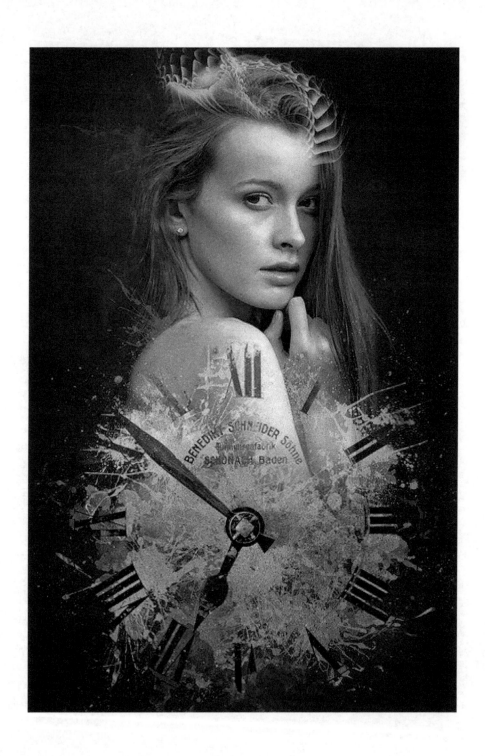

Everything Started with a Headset

In these times it is common to see a young person glued to a cell phone. Always watching social networks, talking with friends, having video calls, living the youth. Although Mia didn't see her son doing that.

Since he was young, he had a cell phone so that they could talk when he was at school. That way she could be sure that in an emergency the little one would take out the device and call. He was never addicted to nets, nor was he ever glued to the phone unless it was for an important call or an online class.

Mia was in favor of not giving her son a cell phone because this was for adults. When she decided to give her son one, it was because one day they were late on the bus and it was a terrible fifteen minutes while the yellow transport was arriving and she knew that a tire had burst. No need to be alarmed. The next day she gave him a cell phone to call in an emergency. She gave it to him with all the rules, that it was a phone for emergencies, not for playing, that he could not take it out whenever he wanted, and that the device was useful, not a toy.

This was inoculated in the young man who, when he grew up and could have been allowed to play on the mobile and be in networks, did not do it, on the contrary, he decided to watch books or at most listen to a podcast or watch a documentary. He was a talented young man and Mia was proud of him.

He had become fond of a lot of cultural content. So, around his 15th birthday, he asked for headphones as a gift so that he could hear better and also study some sounds to create musical scores. Mia proudly set out to find the best for him.

She found some of Chinese brand but they promised to have everything and a very clean sound, the Chinese who sold them to her said in very bad English that if the son did not like them, he would take them to her and she would surely change them and even pay for the inconvenience. Mia found the way in which the Chinese man guaranteed her headset so convincing that she chose them.

A few days later it was the young man's birthday and he was looking forward to his presents. Each of the family members gave him their gifts, not to mention the aunt's awful socks, a games console he already had from another uncle, a couple of books he wanted from a cousin, and finally the most desired gift. The one his mother was going to give him. He opened the special package and found a box with the headset printed in Chinese letters.

-It wasn't the brand I asked for, Mom. -said the annoyed young man.

-I know, but where I looked for them the salesman told me that you would like these better, if you don't like them tomorrow we'll go get the others.

The young man made a gesture characteristic of his age and opened them, they were a red headset opaque as the color of clotted blood, powerful, with a thick wire and a number of options. He looked for the cell phone and put the connector on it. He put the headphones on his ears, adjusted them to the size of his head, typed something into the cell phone, and opened his eyes wide when he started to listen. His face was a pleasure like his mother had never seen before.

-Are they good? -Mia asked, knowing the answer in advance.

-"They're amazing," he said, looking at the others at the table and saying, "Excuse me."

He gets up and goes to his room. After a while, he looked over to say goodbye to the others because his mother had forced him to, but it seemed that he just wanted to have the headset hugging his ears.

That night she didn't see him anymore. The next day he went downstairs, with the device on his head and the cell phone in his hands. What he had never done before was now beginning. He seemed to be out of date.

-Good morning," his mother says.

-As soon as he answered, he seemed out of it.

Mia didn't mind, she knew her son, he had always been a young man who wasn't addicted to anything, she assumed he was lost in his music, connecting and adapting, they were his first headset, what could it hurt? The days went by and the rituals that Mia and her son had were broken, they no longer ate dinner together as they did every day, because her son always had something to do in the room. On the weekends, they didn't play scrabble like they used to because the son composed the best song ever made.

The most curious thing of all is that he always had his headset, they were an extension of his head. Although he didn't have the hostile attitudes of age, he was as out of it as any teenager who enjoys his cell phone, only in this case it was the headset that had him lost.

In the second month, Mia began to worry. One night she went to the bathroom and saw a glow under her son's door, she opened it carefully, hoping not to attract her son's attention, while opening it she regretted it, thinking she might find her son touching himself while watching some erotic video, she almost closed it, but she remembered that she had just seen the clock and it was 3:05 in the morning. Her son was on his cell phone, his eyes were wide open and he didn't seem to see the device, what he seemed to be doing was listening.

-You turn that off and go to sleep right away. -she ordered him.

Her son jumped up, didn't expect to see her there, took off his headphones, and saw his mother, detailing her. As if she had time without being there. He nodded and walked to bed. He went to bed and fell asleep immediately. Without saying a word.

Mia looked at the headset for a while, put them on a sofa in her room, and went out to sleep. Her son woke up the next day as good as new, he looked like his old self, he was talkative, he even listened with surprise to stories that Mia had told him days before and it seemed that he had never heard them.

The rest of the day they talked and shared, when night fell, the young man took the headphones again, when Mia saw that he was going to connect again she said

-With control, that I have seen you very addicted to that thing, remember that in this house we have to control the vices.

-Yes, Mom, I know.

If before the situation had been worrying, now it was worse, as soon as your son put on his headset, it was as if he had disconnected from the world, he was present but at the same time absent. She typed and stayed long enough to pay attention to what was being heard in the headset. Mia spoke to him twice and didn't utter a word, barely nodding his head as if to imply that he had heard and was now out of the way.

Mia didn't give it much thought that day, she went to sleep and the next day was a working day again. In the evenings she arrived, greeted her son, and talked a little with him, although he seemed not to be present, he was lost in that headset again. Mia did not want to think badly, she hoped it was just a stage, like so many stages that young people go through. All this changes one day when she gets a call from the school, they wanted to know if her son was okay, he hadn't been going to school for weeks, precisely since after his birthday, he was one step away from losing the whole school year.

That day Mia realizes that she is facing a real problem. She talks to her boss and goes home early, takes her car and goes on the gas to get there fast, she was full of a lot of anger and in turn, her brain was confused, the behavior was not characteristic of her son, on the way she thought it might be the fault of some woman who had seduced him, and he was floating in love and had forgotten his responsibilities.

She also thought it might be the fault of drugs, he was at the age to smoke pot or inject things, although this ruled out, and her son would not even go out.

All sorts of guesses went through her mind and she knew in every one of them that it was the headset that was to blame, the one that had brought out a side of her son that she did not know.

When she got home, she went in so quickly that the front door was left open. Mia shouted her son's name, got no answer, ran upstairs to the room, and there the door was ajar. Inside was her son, on the sofa, wriggling, with his feet dragging, looking lost, as if he were on drugs. She approached him, took off his headphones and the young man seemed to return, as if he had woken up.

Mia shouted at him, complaining that he had dropped out of school, that he was in a lot of trouble and would have to go to school the next day. The young man said nothing, he was dazed, it seemed that all the accusations were new to him.

Mia smelled the atmosphere and realized that he hadn't even bathed, so she sent him to clean up with the threat of a beating if he didn't go immediately.

The young man ran to the bathroom and Mia stared at the headset he still had in his hands, thought about it for a few minutes, and then put them in her ears. She felt the comfort of the foam in her ears, they were nice. As soon as she did so, it was as if she had teleported, felt a pleasure she had never experienced before, sat down where her son had been minutes before, and let herself go.

No one noticed that the connector on the hearing systems was not connected to anything. Her son's cell phone was unloaded under the pillow.

A Working Woman

She met her husband when they were just 19 years old. She fell madly in love from the first day and liked every act her husband had, filled her up, loved the man very much, and showed it to her at all times.

He seemed to be a good man, attractive, pleasant, with a gift to please everyone. He smiled with a smile of white teeth carefully cared for by his mother.

This caused Bonnie a love and adoration for this man that at the time was noticed by her parents and also by her friends. Even one of her best friends, Aby, withdrew her friendship when she noticed that Bonnie would not listen to her. She told her that she could no longer be friends with a woman who could not see beyond her nose, and that adoration of a man did not go with her.

Bonnie took it as a betrayal, when on many occasions she had heard her lovers' dislike, now she could not enjoy being in love with her. Selfish, that's what she thought. At that time she didn't give it much importance because she was in love with her partner and even more so when he went to the house and with the greatest formality in the world officially asked for her parents' hand in marriage.

Later his parents felt honored that such a beautiful woman from a good family was chosen by their son to share his life. The two were married in the eyes of God on April 19 in a small church and only with their families, this at the request of the groom, who said it was so they could have an intimate space where no one would bother them and they would be comfortable sharing only with their loved ones.

They traveled to Niagara Falls for their honeymoon, hugging and sailing in the boat where they saw the waterfall. Bonnie was thrilled, watching the couples declare a thousand and one ways and she was standing next to her new husband.

They stayed in a modest hotel, but she didn't care, because from the moment they arrived the man brought out his dominant side, something that excited her and she let herself be loved in the thousand and one ways he asked her to, as a good wife and willing, she gave in to many games she enjoyed, some even with a little pain, but it didn't matter, all to please him.

So she felt totally connected to him and on that honeymoon, one of the best moments of her life, they made the first child, who was born nine months later. During the pregnancy, the man treated her very well, indulged her every whim, spoiled her, and when the little one was born he behaved like the best father of all.

Bonnie was always by her little one's side and when her husband asked her to travel somewhere to try out business, she went, for her everything was her husband, for him whatever it took, until the end of the world, to a collapsing Chilean mine, to the Amazon to extract gold or to the bottom of a burning volcano. Together until death.

During one of those trips, she became pregnant with her second child, this time a female was born, with whom her husband broke up, she was his princess and he took her wherever he went.

14

He filled her with many gifts, spoiled her, and was a great father. The little girl felt lucky to have her father so attentive to her and he allowed himself to be spoiled as well.

To the outside eye, they were the typical American family, the woman with the short hair, settled in the beauty parlor that morning, the children playing happily, the husband with a cigarette in his mouth, reading the newspaper with his legs crossed, the dog jumping up and down to the rhythm of the children's games and a white railing outside with the grass finely cut.

As the years passed, the couple settled in like any other, with routines, accepting the good and bad in each other, going out for walks every now and then, and dealing with the growth of the two children who soon arrived at high school and were considering college. They had been living in the same house for years, and it wasn't long before the couple would be alone when the young men took a trip to college. The first one to leave was the boy and soon after the daughter, both good, obedient children who were happy to leave their mother's womb to live their lives. Some time after the children leave and the couple lives alone in that house that seems to be getting bigger than ever. One day the husband seems to be sick, he started with a severe fracture that followed with a vomit of blood that forced them to go to the hospital. He had stomach cancer that had spread to his liver. A few months later the man died, becoming one of the family men who would be forgotten in the next generation.

Bonnie was left alone and felt helpless, as a child would feel when abandoned by his mother in a terminal. Not knowing where to go. She spends a few days in this grief of being left without her husband, who for many years was the love of her life.

Being a widow, she began to think about her past years, and a desire was born to get to work on something that would give her life meaning. So she enters one of those pyramid-shaped companies, where she starts at the top and takes advantage of it to recover those friends from the past, to call them to go for a coffee and offer them to enter the business.

Bonnie looks like another one, because she looks confident, she looks independent, her children are surprised because that woman had not always been the shadow of their father. Now she was someone who without a commitment to children or a husband was doing something for herself after so many years.

She quickly grows within the company and her income becomes juicy, although what she is least interested in is money, what she likes is to feel alive, active, achieving things that she never could in her life.

One afternoon, while she was at home drinking coffee from her husband's cup, she put out her hand and let go of the cup. Even with coffee in it, it fell and shattered, spilling the liquid all over the floor. She had just realized something: she hated her husband.

She hated him from the first moment they were married, when she began to notice that the man was never as loving as she dreamed. They went on their honeymoon to the place where he should have asked her to marry him and not in his car, taking the ring out of her pocket and performing the ritual with annoyance.

Nor should he have subjected her to his first sexual encounter to acts that are asked of a prostitute, so many new things in so few days in a fleabag motel.

She couldn't stand so many trips, so many changes in her life and in the end when they settle down it's in a house that he liked but she hated, neither could he ever be in the places that she wanted so much, she always had to go to his side and her dreams were forgotten for years.

When he became ill she should have been by his side, until he finally took his last breath and with this, the chains he had put on her for twenty years were over, she was free and happier than ever.

That day she didn't even dry the coffee that later became a sticky stain, nor did she pick up the broken cup. She went into the bedroom, took out her husband's clothes, made a pile of them, and set fire to them in the garage, along with all the things that were meaningful to the man. She didn't want to have anything of his in the house, she just wanted to forget him, something difficult, but it was clear that the chains had been broken forever, she was free as ever.

From then on Bonnie recovered her lost youth, she looked less years old than she really was and was a working woman who enjoyed every day. Soon she was one of the most admired in the company where she worked and she climbed to high levels. She was there until the day she died, where dozens of people fired her and remembered her for many years.

She did have a meaningful life.

Finding Love

Callie was looking for love since she was young. She was always a romantic woman. When she first entered school, she was enthralled with the boy she liked so much and when they went out to play she gave him a kiss, he was another boy just like her. The little boy was frightened, as it usually happens with men when a woman shows interest

That's how it happened to her throughout her life. When she was in school, she made out with some boys who took her for an easy woman, because she was always looking forward to getting a real boyfriend.

Even as a teenager the boys were looking for her because they hoped to get a second base with her. When Callie liked a boy, she would show it by giving him some kisses and let his hands go through spaces that she had not had before. Her breasts were then pawed by many and some more daring boys, who, in the midst of the passion, would put their hands in her crotch, but there her modesty would jump up and down.

Time went by and finally when she was about to graduate, the field marshal put his eye on her, he was the man she had always wanted, in the middle of the party they had, drunk both of them, he took her to one of the rooms and after a few morbid words he stripped her and they had quick sex that was far from what a girl expects for her first time, painful, without subtlety and with the bitter taste that remains when it is a meaningless sex. Callie, far from feeling the pleasure she expected, was depressed and went home, where she cried for a whole day without clearly understanding what was going on.

Every person is born with a desire that they want to achieve no matter what, for some reason Callie was always in love, she could never be described as a slut because she was not, she never cheated on anyone and her mind only ran with totally innocent thoughts where she wanted a man to tell her that he loved her and to go with her like all those soap opera stars that had taken so many sighs from her.

But this type of love did not end up arriving, she did not have that boy she wanted, who sighed with her, who wrote her love poems, who sang songs to her with an off-key voice, who looked at her and even begged her for a little love. Callie was very dreamy, always thinking of all kinds of scenes where the boys looked at her with their little eyes of a slaughtered sheep and asked her for a kiss and she would beg, but in the end, she would jump to hug and kiss them.

She had a subscription to wedding magazines and she knew all the variety of models, the best in the market and what the princess of such a country had worn for her wedding and she imagined herself in that dress with her beautiful dress next to it and on the altar, receiving God's blessing.

But it did not happen, that desperation to find love had made her a victim of comments, the neighborhood whore, that whoever came to seduce her could have her and in part it was true, what many ignored was that she was opening her heart every time she received one of these men and hoping to be reciprocated just as she did with them.

There is no evil that is there causing harm that does not end up generating a scale in the person. This is what happened to Callie, who got tired of having those kinds of men in her life who only showed up to put her to bed, and when they satisfied their desire, they didn't return her calls. Then she began to feel a resentment towards men that became more aggressive, more painful every day. Even when a man came with lewd intentions, she looked at him with disgust and did not accept. She had her weak days where she would allow someone to seduce her and go to bed with him, but then she would throw him out herself before giving way to harm.

She would sigh in her loneliness, wishing she could have the opportunity to be loved, she would deny her pain because the loved one was not there, but she would not allow anyone to notice, even in the neighborhood people would comment that now she was not seen with anyone, some men would say that they had tried to seduce her but without luck and this was a joke because if a man was not able to take Callie to bed, it was very bad to seduce.

But they soon realized that she was another one, that she didn't want to continue being the talk of the town, that she couldn't take another insult from some woman who called her a slut because she had slept with her boyfriend or worse, her husband. But Callie hadn't even noticed that the man was engaged, for her the man who appeared with seductive intentions, was because he was free and wanted something serious.

You may think she had a screw loose, but no, she was an extremely intelligent, hard-working, professional woman and had even known how to knead money, only that she found it a bit difficult to understand the sharp or dark sides of love, that not everything was like soap operas and that love was far from what you saw in Disney cartoons.

So, from being an easy woman to pick up, who with four sentences would go with the guy, she had now become an airtight woman who saw any man's approach as a threat.

Morgan was a long-time colleague of Callie's, and he witnessed her hanging out with several men from the company and then greeting each other as if nothing had happened. She never looked at Morgan with any other intentions, and he watched her in silence without even paying her a compliment, even though he was taken with her from the first day he saw her.

He liked the woman very much, she was attractive, smiling, kind, and intelligent and he felt a strong attraction as he had never felt with any woman, the only thing he felt like a weight, was that she behaved like a slut and seemed to have no self-respect that stopped his advances to seduce her.

Although he felt relief when he heard in the corridors that she was rejecting men and that now she wanted to adopt an attitude of dignity, as if they did not know her.

Morgan felt a slight burning when he heard these derogatory comments. One day, when he feels up to the task, he approaches Callie and they talk about work, the weather, and anything else. He looks for a way to ask her out. When he told her, the woman changed her attitude and looked down on him.

—I could have expected it from anyone, but you, Morgan? What a disappointment.

Then she walked away and left him there, bewildered and not understanding what had happened.

A few weeks passed and again Morgan had the opportunity to talk to her, after setting the mood he told her.

—I don't know what you understood the other day, I would never want to hurt you, I didn't mean to offend you.

—I didn't mean to offend you. I'm sure you do, like everyone here, you have a fixation on me, if you want to empty your testicles, go to a brothel, use your hand, I'm nobody's toy.

Morgan was going to try to explain himself, but the woman came out at a fast pace and left him with the word in his mouth.

Some time later he approached her and went to the point, with sincerity.

—I've liked you ever since you went out with your friends, ever since I saw everyone saying bad things about you that I tried not to hear, I've always liked you. I never dared to say anything to you because I wasn't the Callie I wanted, despite the strong attraction I had for you. But now, where everyone comments that you reject them, that you walk alone, in search of yourself, I am even more attracted to you and my intentions to go out with you is to get to know you better, not to get you into bed, I care about you, what you are, not your body. I like you, Callie.

The woman looked at him, moved, but without saying anything, she put her hand on his shoulder and left.

That night at home, Callie's head was a whirlwind, she thought about all that Morgan had told her and that he seemed to be what she had always looked for, she thought about him and she had never seen him as a prospect, but she thought that he was not bad, that she could accept a coffee from him, talk to him, get to know him a little.

The next day, she was the one who looked for him and told him to have a coffee.

When they left work they had a coffee far from the stress of the office and began to feel that they had many things in common and that they were comfortable, little by little they got to know each other better and formed a stable relationship, an idyllic love as Callie had always wanted. Love had finally found her, when she had stopped looking for it as a desperate person.

The Breakthrough of Perfection

She's looking at the ceiling, that white, polished ceiling that her husband arranged so carefully. Now he is an orphan, as is she, the new widow. Since she died her dream has not been the same, but how can it be if for thirty years you slept with the same man by your side. The love of life, with whom you first shared a bed. When they were young and fiery, they gave themselves up and felt their skins; when love calmed down to give way to a more leisurely relationship; when they went to bed angry, and even when they had that lover with whom they almost left the house and when they made up, they lived a sort of second passion.

The bodies deteriorated in bed, fatter, with less smooth skin, wrinkles, and aches. It is known that at some moment one of them will leave this world, but this is as hard as saying goodbye to the mother, one knows that someday she will die, but to accept that she is not the woman full of life and now she is an old woman, it is very difficult to accept that that side of the bed will be empty forever.

How love hurts. Even if you live with a couple for many years, finally the sunset comes where one leaves and the other ends up crying about the departure of this one or giving thanks because he left, everything depends on how it was.

In this case, Celia, our protagonist, misses her husband very much, she feels that the bed is itching, that she is hot and that she is immersed in an ocean of mattress, that the bed is too big for her.

She gets up, puts on her slippers, feels them too hot on her feet, and walks barefoot, feels the ice cream on her soles, and is relieved by it because she is hot.

She goes to the closet, opens the door and sees her husband's side, there are finely arranged all the suits she wore during her life as a married man and businessman, clothes made to measure, perfection, the man was perfect, a whole picture, a real gentleman, he fell in love with her the old-fashioned way and never failed except for the time of the crisis when he fell in love with another woman, but he was always a man who respected her, who never spoke to her in a bad tone and even his anger was in style.

Years as manager of his own company, he knew how to educate his children with discipline, with tenacity and made them good people who also managed to reach the highest levels of quality. In front of her, she had the remains of a man as few are born in this world, and how she missed him, how she felt the weight of absence.

She noticed this every morning when she served an extra cup of coffee and then remembered that her husband was not there, she threw the cup in the sink and cursed her luck. She said that she should have died first, not her husband, although later she thought about how she would have taken it and surely she would have fallen into a depression and suffered more, because that is what Celia had, that although she suffered, she was brave, she was tough and did not break down so easily, her husband, although he was brave, on an emotional level sometimes broke down before her, and this blow surely she would not have endured.

Two weeks after her husband's death there was a knock at her door. When she opened it was a young man with a FedEx T-shirt holding a box in his name that was already paid for.

Celia signed for it and took the box, saw that the sender was her husband, was very surprised to see her husband's name on it, opened the package with trembling hands and hurled some insults at the shipping company for closing the packages with such dedication.

When she finally removed the wrapping she had a small wooden box in front of her that had paper inside. She opened it and put her hand to her mouth, because she almost started to cry. He began to pass the papers one by one, everyone knew them, they were already worn out by the years, but they were those, his love letters, many of those she wrote for him, wrappings of knick-knacks, photos of when they were young with signatures behind each other. The many details that the two of them gave each other when they were engaged and in the spring of their marriage, each one of the details, was such a dedication with which he had kept her, that many did not even remember them as much as he remembered them. When she finished checking everything, she found a new sheet of paper, which looked recent, had her husband's shaky handwriting, written in black pen.

Dear and beloved Celia, I am starting to write these letters with a lot of pain, because I know that if you read them it is because I am already dead.

Life was so cruel that it took me first than you and now you are alone. I'm sure you are surprised by this box you received, but let me tell you that all this time I have kept it with the love I have had for you since day one and I hope that on the other side of life I have them too or that I live like a loop the wonderful love story you were.

You are the best thing I had in life, you who gave me the other wonderful gift, our children, I love you very much, and I hope from the other side to protect you and watch over your dream.

I love you. Don't forget to drink the chamomile water with plenty of Stevia so you can sleep and don't suffer from insomnia, even more so now that you're upset about my death, which I know you, when you're stressed out you don't sleep.

All-day long she read the letter and reviewed every detail the husband had put in it, the story of a love narrated in letters and details of decades of marriage. Everything or had saved what man keeps those memories? This was not the only thing, because a week and a half later they played at her place again, this time it was a florist company that brought her an immense bouquet full of pink flowers and coves, they made the arrangement as if it was a swan and her husband was the sender.

When she unfolded the leaf, it said in his handwriting:

Happy anniversary, my beautiful, such a day as there is we got married and it was the moment I was happiest in life. I hope that at this moment you have by your side this arrangement of flowers made just as I asked, the pink flowers as you always liked, the coves you loved so much and the swan that was the symbol of our love, and that united us forever since we were young, when we knew that swans once in a couple, is for all life

Not even death will be able to untie the love I feel for you and my demonstrations of this eternally for you. I miss you, I don't know where I am now, but I know that from where I am, I miss you.

Celia felt bad, guilty, because she had forgotten the anniversary, she was going to fold the sheet, but she realized that in a fold there was a message for her.

PS. I know that at this moment you will feel guilty because you didn't remember our anniversary you never did, it was the joke of our love, I sometimes forgot it. Right now you are forgiven because it should not be difficult to deal with my death, so do not feel guilt about it, on the contrary, feel happiness that today in our day, you have before you those beautiful flowers that will remind you how much I love you.

Celia smiled bitterly and knew that her husband knew her more than anyone else, even after his death.

During the following days she took care of protecting the flowers so they would not die so soon, when her death was inevitable she took a cove and a rose and kept it folded with the letter, to keep that beautiful bouquet in mind, she also took a photograph so she could contemplate it as much as she wanted.

For several weeks her husband did not manifest himself, but she knew that soon she would have another detail. Her birthday was coming up. That day, at noon, while the children were at home, sharing their birthday with her, there was a knock at the door, when she opened it, some mariachis started singing with a man with a beautiful voice. When the song ended, the mariachi said that it was a present from her husband who from beyond wished her a happy birthday.

It was a bittersweet serenade that had one more detail at the end. The only woman in the mariachi band came up to her, took off her huge hat, and handed her a letter with a sealed envelope.

—This is what your husband leaves you, he sends you to say that he will love you forever and he is waiting for you on the other side.

She gave her a kiss on the cheek. Celia felt her cold lips and was left with the feeling that she had left lipstick on her skin.

With her index finger she caressed the hard texture of the sealing wax, she always took pleasure in these stamps. They looked so elegant. She opened the letter with trembling hands and took out the sheet, unfolded it, and began to read.

Happy birthday my wife.

By now the mariachis must have already sung, I looked for the best one of all. One that you always praised me, I hope they sang as they suggested in their advertisements. Love, this is the last letter I will send you, I think the previous ones and these left a painful taste and I do not want you to suffer, enough with my absence.

The purpose of these letters was that you could keep in mind that it doesn't matter anything, from where I am I love you and I protect you, just as I had in mind to give you all the details that you have received, I also took care of every detail, you will never lack anything, not even me, because from here I protect you.

The letters I gave you and the details were to remind you of the beauty of our marriage, so that you will remember the beauty and not get caught up in my death.

Finish enjoying what you have left of life, that when God calls you, here I will be waiting for you on the other side.

Always yours...

Her older son sat down next to her and stroked her back

—What's going on, Mom? —he asked, worried.

—Nothing, son, everything is fine, only even if one does not want it, the end of perfection always comes.

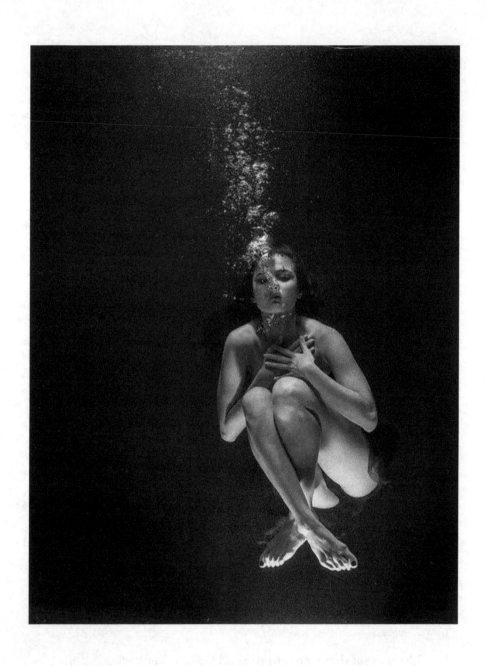

The Burden of All

From: Cadence <CadenceM@gumal.com>

Date: Mon, 7 February 20 at 7:32

Hello friend. How I miss you, I'm missing a lot to talk with you and to be able to connect to tell you all the changes I'm suffering now. In the last email, I told you how I'm doing with my pregnancy. Uff, the last few months were terrible, I was throwing up every day, I had cravings and a mood where I hated Roger all the time.

I feel immensely happy, seeing him there, that little thing that came out of me, that sees me with those little eyes full of so much innocence, that smiles at me and loves me, that gurgles out words and I want him to say mommy.

That little being has changed my life and you can't imagine how happy I feel right now. All I need is you, to be able to listen to you, to be able to tell you so much, and for you to tell me that I am a romantic to die for and that at some time it is telling you that being a mother is a cross.

I don't believe how this beautiful little thing could be a cross. Although I confess that ten minutes ago I felt my hand full of something slimy, it was the baby's poo, no matter how much soap and water I poured on it, the smell doesn't seem to go away.

Write, my friend, that sometimes you forget about the poor beings, of course, as you are in Paris, seducing Frenchmen and drinking wine, since we don't even write to the poor newborn. Ungrateful.

With love... Cadence.

.

From: Cadence <CadenceM@gumal.com>

Date: Mon, February 27 at 9:30

Hello friend. I've had a rough month, the baby made green poop and was also spending sleepless nights. He didn't sleep at all, so the next day I had huge dark circles under my eyes and he was sleeping divinely.

Not to mention how my tits are on fire from all that baby sucks and you're going to tell me that he's a little boy, that he's going to hurt me if he doesn't even have any teeth, well he does, it's like he's going to rip my nipple off.

I've also spent a few days where I get very depressed, I don't know why. Although I'm better now, I'm getting better, the pediatrician told me that my depression was part of the hormones.

We are complicated. I liked the photos you sent me from Paris, send others.

I miss you.

From: Cadence <CadenceM@gumal.com>

Date: Mon, 12 March at 15:30

Hello friend. Thank you for what you say about the baby, yes, he is beautiful, at least he doesn't look like his dad who looks like a coconut, he is handsome my prince, I feel like eating him with kisses.

I'll tell you a secret, sometimes I see him sleeping, he has several hours like that and I miss him, I wake him up gently and when he starts crying I lull him to sleep and devour him with kisses.

Although surely this is what all mothers do.

With love.

Cadence.

From: Cadence <CadenceM@gumal.com>

Date: Mon, December 24 at 7:32

Merry Christmas, my friend, Santa Claus is coming home tonight, the boy still doesn't understand about it, but we bought him a big cuddly toy of a cat, which he loves. Besides clothes and details to make him happy. This year of so many challenges and so many things is already closing, Jeff who went to Afghanistan, the baby who has taught me so many things, work, Roger, in short, everything we have suffered and enjoyed. But today is not the day to be thinking about those things, but to enjoy and be happy for the times to come. I am honored to have you as a friend and again, it is another Christmas without your presence. Without you by my side.

I miss you, I wish you a Merry Christmas. Don't get drunk, as always.

Merry Christmas.

From: Cadence <CadenceM@gumal.com>

Date: Mon, March 20 at 8:10

Friend, the prince started to walk, we all got excited here, he put on his two little feet, shaking, with a huge laugh because he knew what a feat he was doing and then he took some quick steps. Running and arriving at my side, we all applauded him.

Now he's walking all over the place, holding on to what he can, like someone who can't swim and is inside a pool.

Here is the video we recorded for you to see.

From: Cadence <CadenceM@gumal.com>

Date: Mon, July 16 at 4:32

This boy is already over two years old, and since he absorbs that boy, he runs all over the house, but of course, since he learned to say some words, he starts screaming like crazy.

Sometimes I ask him to calm down because there comes a point when I can't stand his screaming. Does that make me a bad mother?

I love my son, but some days he overflows. I feel that I need a break, I go into the bathroom, and soon after he shows up there, knocking on the door with his little hand, he doesn't want anything, just to be pampered or to show me something. He already starts to show spoiled behavior.

That child promises, he has character.

PS. About what you told me, yes, your boyfriend is an idiot, you shouldn't have let him do that to you. In your shoes, I would leave him to learn.

From: Cadence <CadenceM@gumal.com>

Date: Mon, May 05 at 3:21

The little one is already in school, he looked beautiful in his academy clothes, incredible that he is already three years old. Not long ago I had him in my arms and he fit in my forearm, small and beautiful. Today he is a little man who says No to everything, and before that, he used to say "why" every time I explained something to him.

Being a mother is incredible, but some days I despair of not being able to do many things or that the child is not as idyllic as it appears in the diaper ads. But I love my child. I love him with my soul. He is my life.

When will you have your child?

Look, you're going to run out of those eggs.

From: Cadence <CadenceM@gumal.com>

Date: Mon, 5 February at 7:32

My child is already 7 years old, how these creatures grow without one realizing it. The truth is that I am surprised with this child who is now a little man and many times I have to get hard in order to face him. He has his character.

A few weeks ago I spanked him because he said a bad word to me, I promised him that the other one would be in his mouth. He has to learn to respect his mother.

It has been difficult, this motherhood, because you start thinking sometimes, children are the best thing in life, but then you sacrifice so much, you leave dreams to be fulfilled, I think that when I am older I will be able to take out of the drawer of memories everything that I could not do now.

From: Cadence <CadenceM@gumal.com>

Date: Mon, 14 June at 9:26

I know what it's like to have a teenager. It is terrible. Today he told me to go fuck myself, yes, like that. That child that I gave birth to, in pain, broke me in half. He told me to go to hell and he did it with rage, with rejection. As if he hated me.

Could it be that he hates me?

That's not all, he has days with a bad attitude, Roger tells me that it's part of the age and that he has his character, that adolescence is difficult, but what mother is prepared for a son to say something as horrible as that. I don't think any. I can't stand so much pain and I can't handle this.

I'm in my day, so everything affects me more, it hurts and I feel that my son doesn't love me. Could it be that he doesn't love me anymore?

We don't even talk anymore, I remember when he was eight years old, less than five years ago, when we were at the table, sitting, talking about everyone as if we were best friends, now? At this moment I am his number one enemy, that child no longer cares about me. To him, I am just a simple general who asks him to do chores around the house and to do his homework. That makes me an enemy.

As soon as I begin my adolescence, what years await me. This child is going to kill me.

From: Cadence <CadenceM@gumal.com>

Date: Mon, 31 August at 10:38

I am writing to you worried, my dear friend. I was putting away the boy's underwear and I found a joint, a big joint about six inches long, to take a few puffs.

I remembered our youth when we smoked our own joints, but I never imagined finding my son doing the same thing, I guess it's the law of life. But now, thinking like a mother, I have my alarms on, because I imagine my boy with an injection machine and his face missing because he injected meth.

This afternoon when he arrives I will talk to him, to tell him that he has to stop smoking, for sure it will be a difficult fight, because he is getting worse every day.

The saddest thing is that my husband doesn't want to support me, it reminds me that we both smoked and we did worse. It's true, it's karma, but I'm sorry, I won't be quiet when I can read the letter to my son so he can stop thinking about doing drugs and ruining his life.

It's already 16 years of this young man, there are two years left and he will be an adult, how I wish I had that little baby, that the worst thing that could happen to him was that he would have a shitty ass. Nothing else.

Being a mother is a gift of life, but also a punishment.

Are you never going to give birth? Not anymore, you married that rich Frenchman who didn't want kids. You were really smart.

Cadence.

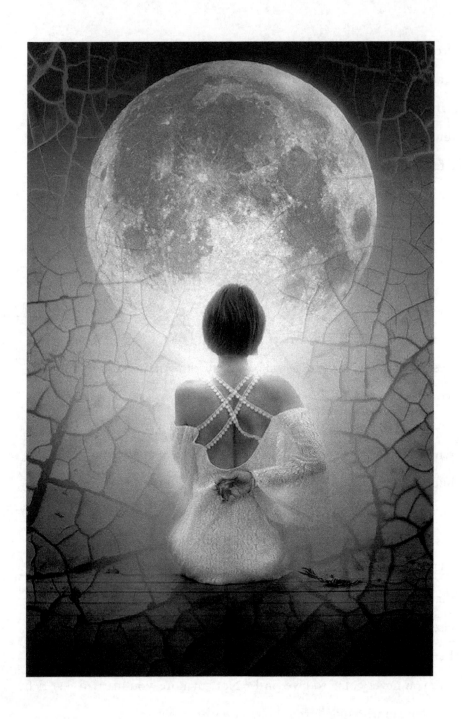

My Lover

I don't remember when we met, I just know that one day we were talking like two acquaintances who want to know each other more.

It happened on Facebook, he appeared on my account and greeted me one day, then he told me something else and then we talked constantly, little by little the hints came out and then we met in person, in a shopping center that was some distance away from each other and that was quite lonely. There we gave each other some delicious kisses, that I do remember, our first kiss, sitting on a bench in the mall, we looked to the sides where no one could see us and we devoured each other, I felt the hot blood of that brown woman, because her tongue ran down the mine and moved like a snake inside my mouth.

That day my hormones were raging, I wanted to take her to a hotel. Although she didn't want to.

From that day to the second date nothing was missing, we met in another part of the city, took a cab and there we went talking about everything a little bit, as if we were going to a business meeting and not to a hotel to get to know each other naked.

When we entered the hotel, we chose a themed room with a round bed and a dome that showed the stars at night. With a bathtub on top where we could get in.

She is the most beautiful woman I have ever loved. So in our first meeting I was very nervous, she kissed me, and started to undress me little by little, she went through parts of my body that I don't want to name here, but that you will have no trouble imagining. Her tongue was not only good at kissing, her expertise made my fear go away. So that day we did it there, but for some reason, I had a resistance that made me repeat with her six times, as if I were a teenager, we were in the bathtub, in bed many times, on a strange piece of furniture and in a position that we loved, me on the edge of the bed and her on her back carrying the rhythm of everything while we looked at ourselves in the mirror.

That day time seemed to be very short, although I must confess that several times when I was enjoying myself more, the guilt wrapped me up, even in one of those I visualized my son running towards me, greeting me, and my wife also looking at me from afar, but they found me like this, naked making love to this woman and seeing the pleasure in my eyes and my body pearly with sweat.

My lover made me forget that feeling of guilt, massaging my back, and giving me an orgasm where I didn't have one.

We continued to see each other, that day and many others, where we met in any corner and went through each other's bodies as we had learned to know it. Something that makes me feel guilty is that when I go through it I feel something that I have never felt with another woman, I have the pleasure as it does not happen with others and I could make love to her all night long, without any problem.

When I think about it, the guilt corrodes me, it is so much that although we both feel so comfortable, I also feel bad and I distance myself from her, the first time I blocked her from the networks and the cell phone, she called me from many other numbers and at the end, full of anger I insulted her and told her to leave me alone.

I don't understand how she can love me if she knows that she is the lover, that when we are having sex in bed at two o'clock in the afternoon, at night I will go to bed with my wife, with my son, in my home. I would not be able to fall in love with a married woman who at night could be having sex with another man. I would not be able to stand it.

For a few months, I managed to keep that woman away, writing to me about false accounts, discovering her by the way she talked, and blocking her again. Always fearing that my wife would realize the betrayal.

One day, I started to miss it, I regretted having blocked it and I unblocked it. She seemed to realize that, because soon after that, the friendship passed to me and I accepted it. We started talking as if nothing had happened and a couple of days later she asked me why I had left.

I explained to her and she told me that I didn't have to worry, that she knew her position, that she didn't ask me for anything, just that I loved her. How hard is it to be a lover? The temptation won me over and we met again, we did not say why, but the meeting was near a hotel and she arrived in a gray cotton dress that looked beautiful, after talking a little we went to the hotel and there I found her beautiful body with a lingerie that had a bow, to open it as a gift. I unwrapped my gift and enjoyed it to the last drop.

That day I was not at all to blame, the scoundrel made me enjoy it like never before, we rolled around in that bed and moaned.

I didn't say, with her there was no worry of pregnancy, she had two children and was sterilized, so we could do it without fear, she would never have children again.

We were dating for a few months and she was afraid I wouldn't leave her again. Sometimes, when she writes to me and I don't answer her soon, she writes to me with more alarm, that if something happens, that if I'm okay. Then I show up and explain to her why I didn't respond and she seems to come back to life. I feel a little guilty about that, because it hurts me that she is so afraid. I don't want her to feel that I don't love her, because I do, I love her and I wish I could be with her longer.

Our dates are always for sex, just once we met and went to a park that is a few hundred meters from a madhouse, it is a place where no one goes, there we went to a small waterfall where we took off our shoes and felt the water on our feet, fresh, divine. We kissed and felt so much that day that we were dying to go to a hotel. But we didn't, we wanted to repeat that encounter, but the next time we met again we locked ourselves in a hotel to make love. That day was phenomenal. She gave herself away like she hadn't for a long time and we tried so many positions and in so many ways that we were exhausted. When we finished we went to a painting conference that was being given at the Museum of Fine Arts, where as the happiest couple in the world we sat down to enjoy the words of the speaker, smiling mischievously, because nobody knew that a few hours earlier we were moaning with pleasure and asking for more. If you ask me, I think that was the best day of all for us.

Although shortly after I did it again, it happened to me when my wife behaved well with me, I felt that I did not deserve so much love and I sent my lover away again, there as the woman did not understand, I insulted her, I said terrible things, I made her angry and then we fought. Not to speak for months.

Many nights before going to sleep I thought about her and how wonderful it would be to have her in bed right now, but then I would fall asleep and never dream about her.

A year later, when I thought I had forgotten her, we made a date, she gave Me Like to a picture and I told her, so we began to talk and we met again in a sleazy motel where we enjoyed ourselves, but we felt that a connector was missing, that things were not the same, she made me notice it, but we did not go into it in-depth, but were entertained at the moment.

One day, we had a little friction and she spoke to me in a way that was like a balloon bursting, I was totally disappointed, I stopped feeling anything for her and the supposed love I had for her is over, now, if she lives or dies I don't care, although every now and then I log in with a fake account to her Facebook and check her photos and think about how she will be.

Sometimes I imagine I'll walk in and find pictures of her and a formal couple and feel a bitter pill choking me. I wouldn't want her to become a bad taste, it's not for me, because I have my wife, but I wouldn't want it to be for anyone else.

Since I left her, I sleep better, the guilt does not corrode me, before, during our time as lovers I could not sleep, and I woke up. Sometimes in the middle of the night, I would wish for her and calm them down myself, but I never spoke to her again.

Although, a few hours ago I liked a picture of me, one from 9 years ago. I know it's her, it's her way of acting. I'm thinking of talking to her, or maybe not. Although an afternoon full of fire with the fire of her body would do this being good.

The Young Man

She was tired of having to put up with everything her husband wanted to do to her, she had to face every day all sorts of scorn and meet her husband and the smell of cheap, prostitute-like perfume, she said, because no other woman would wear something of such bad quality and much less mess with a married man.

For many years she has put up with a man who has not valued her. She has never lacked anything, she has money, she has comforts at home and she travels whenever she wants. Her husband holds a major political office, in addition to having multi-million dollar businesses. They live in the most exclusive area of the city and with 360-degree panoramic views. That's why Chastity can't stay. She has everything a woman could want, plus she was born in a poor neighborhood and went through hardships before positioning herself as the wife of a businessman, who then used her as a trophy. When she met him, she was just a young girl, and the man was already his age, 10 years different to be exact. She lacked nothing, she was beautiful, with an angelic face, with a mischievous look. But the man who would be her future husband filled her with details, sent her to have surgery, put her breasts, made her increase her buttocks a little bit and operated her nose and other little details, all this with trips, luxuries and the latest in fashion and technology. The young lady from the neighborhood became the lady of the important businessman, who later entered politics.

Few know Chastity's past, for when her husband was known throughout the United States and the world, she was already his mistress. But men, when they have power, want more, so after having his wife safe and giving her everything she wanted, she started looking for other women, mostly young girls.

Chastity fought, made scenes, and took out those neighborhood roots that characterized her, all in order to prove that she was the lady and the others were the bitches. It didn't work, a man with power is arrogant and blind. What moves him is his ego and that is what hurts him most when he is hurt.

That's why she decides to start a plan. She opens a Facebook account where she puts her best picture and starts following a lot of guys. The first few days she talks to several of them and gets nowhere, just talking about typical nonsense that is talked about in networks, little by little she starts to flirt better, she flirts with some guys, but cuts them off when they send her a picture of their member without asking for it. She feels disgusted by this vulgar act. Those romances are behind her and those details of the gentlemen are now so frugal.

Finally, she manages to find a very good-looking young man. He is 22 years old, studying music, white, with pink lips, finely combed hair, easy smile, friendly, with a rich verb, and with a wide culture. His name is Kevin, they start talking and Chastity is captivated by being surrounded by such a gentlemanly man. Besides, at that age, he is very influential and allows himself to be manipulated.

Every night, from her bed, with her silk pajamas and her expensive perfume, alone as always, she began to talk to the man. He was already there, attentive to talk, the hours began to go by and without realizing it, and they were talking at two o'clock in the morning. One night at almost three o'clock, both said they felt a strong attraction. Chastity recognized this, she liked the man, but her intentions with him were different, they were different plans, revenge was what nourished this relationship.

In the chat, she was waiting for a proposal from him.

—Let's meet.

She didn't know what to say, because the photo she had posted was one of those traps, where they showed and didn't show, a profile that didn't allow anyone to guess it was her, but which did show that they were talking to a very beautiful woman.

One night where her husband told her he was going to a business meeting, which she knew was the phrase he used when he wasn't coming back until the next day, Chastity dressed up and met Kevin at the entrance of a shopping mall. She asked him to get in the car, not to meet her outside, because she hadn't confessed to him, but she was a public figure.

That night she put on a red signature dress, and subtly put on makeup, perfume, and her long light brown hair fell down her back. When she parked at the meeting place, Kevin was already there. He, who sensed that she was an important woman, was careful to dress in a suit that didn't fit him but didn't make him look bad either.

The young man entered the car naturally and was surprised for a few seconds, he didn't expect to meet the person inside.

—Is something wrong? —asked Chastity, who was beginning to feel uncomfortable.

—I didn't expect...

—What?

—No, it's nothing bad. When you told me you were an older woman, I imagined a more... mature, older woman, but you're... you're very beautiful. You leave me speechless. You are extremely beautiful, Chastity.

—You're not far behind. You are very beautiful.

They both smiled, she started the car and they hit the road, she didn't say where they were going, but the plan was to go to a retirement home they had outside the city, it was a place her husband never went to, however, when she arrived she stayed a few feet away, confirming that her husband wasn't there with some woman. When she saw no movement, she took out the remote control, opened the garage and they went in.

—What are we going to do here?

—It's a house we have for special moments.

—Wow.

—We'll be very quiet here. I have some wine that you are going to love and we can listen to music, do you want to?

—As long as it's with you, anything.

They get out of the car and go into the house. It was a luxury house, one of those escape houses that have a view of the city and that even though they never visit it, they keep the elegance that only the rich know how to put in the houses.

They talked for a while, but between the two there was already chemistry, they let it emerge at the second glass, when the mouths met and the breaths began to become choppy. She put her cup aside and caressed his face. Kevin felt his hand wet from the perspiration from the cup. He caressed her back and both of them relaxed and stripped off their clothes.

Chastity drowned out several small cries of pleasure that night, as she felt the youth of that man on her, who seemed to feel the most fortunate to be traveling with a woman he said was the most beautiful of all. When they were over she was very happy. It had been a long time since anyone had made love to her, only sex and reluctantly. She already knew that her husband had stopped loving her and had her like a vase.

Today, she remembered all of her femininity and from that night on, the malevolent plan she had to take revenge on her husband, to see if he would wake up and try to get his wife back. But the plans changed, now they started a clandestine relationship where they met at every opportunity to frolic and little by little Chastity also began to fall in love with that young man. Soon, she began to help him pay for his things, like his college, clothes, personal payments, and money to use as he wanted.

She had fallen in love, she had to admit it, and he seemed to feel the same way. This retirement home had become the love nest and now they began to see each other not only at night, but also during the day, the best thing is that they lived in danger, which is what makes everything more exciting.

Chastity began to plan the masterstroke, she asked Kevin for six months to escape, then she began to move capital, a lot of money, she would not leave empty-handed. She placed a few million in accounts that could not be violated by her husband, in tax havens. After a few months, she had enough money to escape and not work another day in her life.

One morning Chastity's husband arrived at the house, as he often did, smelling of a lover and liquor. When he entered, he lay down on the bed and didn't even notice, six hours later when he woke up with a stitch in his head and exhausted, he shouted his wife's name but she never showed up. He became suspicious when he saw the empty closet, there was little left of her in the house. From there he began to investigate, he asked intelligence to look into it and it was not difficult to find Kevin, the conversations and the first date, at which point the connection via Facebook was paused, the husband already knew who Chastity had left with, he followed the bread crumbs and saw that zeros were missing from the account, he continued to snoop around and found out that she had left the country. By the time he came to find out, his wife was already in someone else's bed enjoying the money she had taken with her for retirement.

Neither all the power this man had, nor the political connections, nor his wounded ego were able to find the woman. Somewhere in the world that for security reasons does not reveal itself, Chastity and Kevin enjoy love and money, gilding themselves in the sun and loving each other like no other.

Sometimes happy endings do exist.

Welcome to America

Finally, the boat seemed to see land in the distance. At first, it looked like a small piece of land that showed that on the other side there was hope and fortune, then it looked better, and you could see that there was life in that piece of land, on one side you began to see the figure of a woman with a big robe and a dagger pointing to the sky. Then you would know that it was the Statue of Liberty.

Welcome to America!

Shouted one of the Irish on the ship, one who had befriended one of the sailors and drank rum all the way, and his face was pink with the joy of having drunk the liquor and of arriving at his destination, as if his life was resolved when he got off.

It was the 1920s and a ship full of undocumented Irish were arriving on American soil to get a chance at a decent life. There Bryony came with her family, she was an only child, her father and mother were on the boat, her grandmother had had to leave her, her mother came back from the trip crying because it was a kind of mourning, she would never see her mother alive again and the grandmother, mother had finally sent her off with a serene gaze, as if wishing that the trip would be a path of roses and joy to serve them to move forward, although in the eyes of wrinkled eyelids you could see the deep sadness caused by being separated from her family.

The ship was finally reaching land, Bryony was seasick the first two days of the trip and her guts were empty as soon as they were full, both her father and mother were distressed, but the captain with a laugh told her that she was a newcomer at sea, that she would soon get used to it, the truth is that she was not the only one seasick, half the ship was vomiting on deck, but on the third day practically everyone was used to it.

When they stepped ashore, they were given their cloth bags and stayed there, in the port, looking around, looking for something to do. An officer ordered them to approach a kind of module, where they had a scribe taking data. Each one gave their name and this was changed to a more American name and so they entered the United States officially.

Bryony's father went through his pockets when he was already in town and found some crumpled bills, he didn't have enough money to cover his expenses. He said they barely had enough money to stay in some boarding house.

They were recommended an old hotel at the end of a blind street, and Bryony was disappointed to find that ugly room, moth-flooded wood, a bed that smelled like it had never been washed, and windows that looked dark because they hit a brick wall. The only window overlooking the street was a place where a man repaired cars.

Bryony didn't sleep that night, she hadn't told her parents, but since they had left Ireland it had been difficult for her to sleep. Now, in that new world, she felt the smells of that flophouse hitting her nostrils. She smelled of urine, stale sweaty sheets, and old wood. All this made her nose itchy and she wanted to sneeze. She was not the only one, because her mother, always silent, obedient, sneezed all night long and when

---

Bryony looked at her, she gave her a smile like "everything is fine".

The twelve-year-old doesn't understand it very well, but they spent several nights there, even though they couldn't afford more than one night. The next day, her mother went out for a couple of hours and when she came back she was happy, with a huge bag of bread and juice for the three of them, although her father didn't eat, because he went out to "see what he could get". For the rest of the day, he did not return and Bryony was able to share with her mother and be a little more at ease without the man's authority.

That night her father returned with rosy cheeks and happy, singing Irish songs. Bryony saw her mother whispering things to him, in reproach, and the man far from being angry said to her in a waiting and cheerful voice.

—Stop scolding me woman, I'm celebrating, I've got a job, tomorrow I start.

And so it was, the next day the man left very early, looking bad because it seemed his head was going to explode, but he put on his work clothes and after crossing the door he left whistling. Her mother told her that he had gotten a job in a sawmill, he had to move wood from one side to the other, chop, unload trucks, whatever came out and also the hardest job, it was Irish, the Irish have to pay for the arrival in the United States, if they want the American dream they have to draw blood from the soul to get it.

That boarding house would be the house of the three for a few months, and Bryony's mother was beginning to get tired, because many nights the little one heard how the wife was complaining to the husband that they had to leave, that they could not continue sleeping badly. Since her arrival in America, Bryony slept on several blankets and had her travel bag as a pillow. She didn't sleep much, so being on the floor or in bed didn't matter to her. But apparently, her mother was uncomfortable seeing her in that condition.

The fights became so intense that some nights Bryony would pretend to be asleep so she wouldn't hear the soothing breaths and body movements that ended with some strange sound from her mother or a guttural groan from her father. Bryony was very sad when that happened because she imagined her father hurting her mother, although the next day she saw her mother happy, bright.

Years later she would understand what was going on there.

A few months after his arrival, he announced with much fanfare that he was going to live in a house, a complete house for everyone, that's how it was, it was an apartment in an old building that was not far from the boarding house.

Her mother, shortly after arriving, began to feel strange discomforts, headaches, dizziness, and a great deal of hunger. She hadn't wanted to announce anything, but the prominent belly gave her away, she was pregnant. Bryony was disconcerted and for several days she didn't know how to handle this feeling, in a short time she wouldn't be the child of the house, but there would be a new member, another mouth to feed. Not to mention the house they were in, which had two rooms, her parents' and hers, she would soon have to share. Her reign in those four walls had been short-lived.

Her father celebrated the arrival of the pregnancy and said a phrase Bryony would never forget:

Let's hope it's a boy now.

For some nights Bryony felt guilty about being born a woman, then she felt the haze that maybe her father didn't love her as he should have because she was a girl. This hurt her.

A few months later her mother said she was in severe pain, her father was gone and Bryony had to carry her mother and follow her orders, take a small bag and walk beside her, while the woman nailed her nails to her shoulders. They walked for ten blocks, at a slow pace, sometimes the woman breathed a sigh of relief and walked faster. Finally, they arrived at a hospital and had to wait for two hours until the woman finally left through a doorway into a restricted corridor.

Twelve hours would pass before Bryony heard from her mother, who was another child. She had been born well, weighed 4,200 kilos and her name was Abby, the little sister had arrived.

Her father finally showed up after it was all over and Bryony noticed his happy face looking through the glass at the little girl.

—The boy was not born, but another doll arrived, as beautiful as my first daughter.

After he told her this, he passed his rough hand across her face, in a loving fatherly gesture.

Bryony felt like the luckiest girl in the world. Years later she would understand that it is difficult to understand her parents at that age, with so many commitments, with so many burdens, it is difficult to cope with the burdens of being in a new world, in a place with so many complications and at the same time be a loving father who reminds his children that they are loved.

Bryony started sharing a room in the house at a few months old, which now smelled of baby powder, poopy diapers, and cologne.

The house seemed to light up with the arrival of the new baby, every day there was something new with him, and his father also seemed to be doing well at work, because apparently, they improved his contract, he would earn more, now that he had a bigger family and they could have more luxuries. For one Christmas he arrived with a huge radio that was the company at night so he could entertain himself. They listened to family radio soaps and the news.

That radio would be the same one that would tell the war times, the war stories, and the events that would come in the next lustrums.

Today many generations have followed Bryony, remember her as a loving grandmother with many stories of her arrival in America, some descendants amassed fortunes, others not so much, but she was part of that Irish wave that today makes up the nearly ten million American citizens.

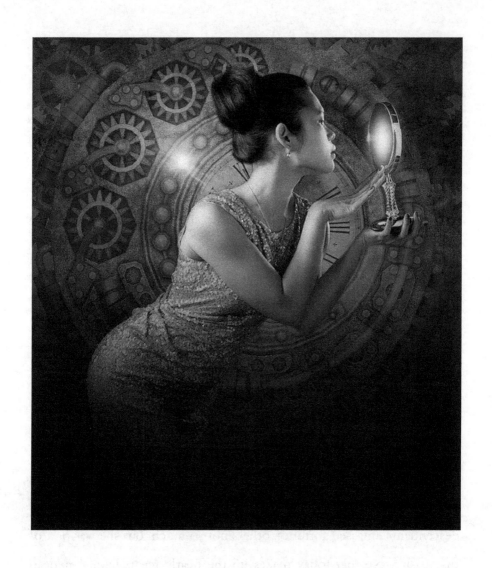

An Ocean in Between

Love has no borders, countries invented imaginary lines in their geographies, but people all the same, except for the ID card that does not differentiate. An act as sublime as love knows it and that is why it manifests itself all the time, as can be seen in the following story.

Two people met in a chat room, he said HELLO, so, in capital letters and she responded in small letters, so they began to know each other and gradually agreed that they liked each other despite the fact that both had very different cultures, and differed in many things, except that they were human beings and felt the same.

Elliot lived in the United States, in the city of San Diego, he was a student of foreign trade, he was 24 years old, he was a gangly young man, skinny, with big glasses and a huge nose, in spite of this description, he was not so ugly, his happy, kind, always positive personality transformed his attitude into someone nice that he attracted in spite of being ugly.

In the United States, he had had a few girlfriends, but because he was so in love, he quickly overwhelmed them and they felt they couldn't continue in that relationship or they might drown.

That's why after a few months or weeks of dating, she would leave him, crying in the corners until a new woman appeared and he would fall in love with her a few days later.

In one of these periods he met his new girlfriend, with whom, although they were not in the same country, they felt a strong attraction and understood each other well.

Internet relationships have a strange good taste that makes you want to stay connected, it's an adrenaline rush of not having the person present, but at the same time, being able to have her so close, just a moment after a message, even though she's on the other side of the world.

The two started with a greeting, with the indifference that starts a conversation in any open chat, but little by little they began to talk about generalities and it seemed that the letters flowed from both sides and soon one asked the other if he had a way they could connect on the outside, a social network, she gave him the email to look for her on Facebook, he did and now they were connected.

There, he began to review her photos and learn more about her personality. He went to information to see if she was in a relationship and breathed a sigh of relief when she announced herself as single.

He saw that she was a very beautiful woman, with her cinnamon color, her black eyes, and her tender and innocent look. Her bushy eyebrows looked like the roof of her eyes that were the lanterns of the beautiful mouth that illuminated the entire face. She was very beautiful, Elliot deduced that at the first moment.

She, Dana, lived in New Delhi, a 14-hour flight from New York, on the other side of the world, in various time zones and many different cultures. She spoke perfect English and he loved getting to know Dana's rich culture. When she saw the HELLO, she responded with the same courtesy she had responded to the other seven guys who were stalking her in the chat room.

But Elliot seemed so nice, that for some reason she did not understand she ignored the other windows and started chatting only with him, then they went to Facebook from where he had a better conversation, of course, she saw some photos and with regret, she realized that he was not the gringo as she imagined him and as she has seen in the movies, but he was not so bad after all.

So, every day they start talking. When one of them wakes up one leaves a message for the other. At six in the evening, Elliot said good morning to Dana, who was just getting up in New Delhi. She wished him good night after he had breakfast. What they agreed on was that they would each get up early in their country so that they could spend some time with each other in the evening so that they could talk a little and deal with the fact that while one was earning his day, the other was sleeping on the other side of the world.

Although it may be a bit far-fetched for people to fall in love even when they are so far away, it created an affection that was more solid than anything they had ever experienced in their lives with people who were physically present.

In one conversation, the inevitable question came up: What are we? What is it that we feel?

The other said: I don't know, but I like it and I don't want to stop.

In this way the two continued to connect, talk, get to know each other a little more each day. Falling in love.

The virtual couple had the first fight one day when they made a video call, she had just gotten up, he was having dinner, and he had a huge burger in his hands.

Dana opened her eyes and watched Elliot chew with pleasure.

—What do you eat? —she asked him.

He looked at the hamburger and said what he was eating, with a tone that made it clear "can't you see?

—What is it?

Elliot responded with a full and casual mouth.

—I don't know. It's meat.

Dana changed her tone, she already knew the answer.

—Meat of what?

—Cow, I guess.

Dana opened her eyes, and with a gesture of annoyance or insult to be more exact, she hung up. Elliot called several times but no luck, no answer. No matter how many times he tried. That night he stayed up until 4 o'clock, trying to get her to answer but no luck.

They would spend several nights where he insisted on writing but she simply didn't want to write back.

It was so much insistence, so much anguish, that finally, Dana answered him. It was she who made the video call and she stayed with a serious face, looking at the camera, as if waiting for an explanation.

—I don't understand what happened. —I don't understand what happened.

—The call is not for an apology, then.

—I apologize, but first I need to know what I did wrong.

—The hamburger that filled your mouth like a beast.

———

66

—Are hamburgers forbidden in India?

—No, but cows are sacred and you called me to show me how you chewed one.

Elliot felt that some extremely valuable information came to him at this time. He remembered that Hindus did not actually kill the cows and understood that he had made the mistake of his life, that he had been a big idiot. He apologized and she forgave him, in those days full of anger she understood that although he had done her a very big offense, it was a cultural contrast that manifested itself.

They returned to the relationship as if nothing had happened, except that Elliot spoke well of the cows on one occasion, saying they were sweet and that he had seen a woman in the field petting one and this one moved affectionately as if it were a spoiled cat.

One day she said she wanted to go to the United States, but that it would be a very complex issue with her parents, he was analyzing his finances, and covering a trip to New Delhi was out of the question for much of his limited income. So they were in limbo as they got to know each other in person.

The months went by in a relationship that although it felt like it was full of a feeling that it had reached the limit that all relationships could reach, the first one that began to feel the consequences was Dana, who one afternoon felt the hairs on her back stand up when she was called by her father and had a brief conversation.

That night she ignored Elliot's messages, the next day they talked, but she was no longer the same, she was distant, she didn't want to tell her boy anything, but she was afraid that he would break when he found out, it was something that sooner or later had to happen.

Elliot helped to speed it up. When he noticed that the attitude had changed, he began to stalk him and ask what was wrong. She finally told him.

—My father is a respected businessman in New Delhi, he knows many powerful and resourceful people. I am his only daughter and what happened was going to happen sooner or later, they asked for my hand, my father has come to an agreement and I am already engaged to a businessman, we have not yet met in person, but I know who he is and we have greeted each other on some occasions. In other words, this thing we have cannot go on, because I would be betraying my future husband.

Elliot had been broken up in many ways, but this was the most prominent of all. He could say that he had been abandoned because his girlfriend had been engaged for cows, goats, and land.

Dana didn't give him much of a chance to beg, when she told him everything and said it was ethical and moral to break up, he said goodbye and told her that he had been special and a few minutes later his hand with a bandage on his thumb, informed Elliot that he was blocked. They had finished.

For a few days he wandered around with his grief, but then he returned to the chat room, now hopefully looking for a woman of his own nationality or Mexican at best.

For her part, Dana, met her husband, he was not the ideal she had, but he was good to her and behaved like a good husband, they had six children and lived with the happiness that any Hindu can have.

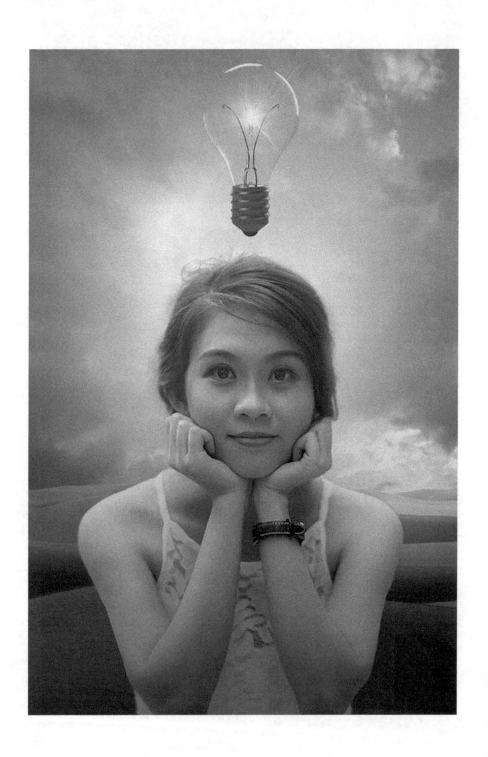

The Unexplained Disease

Diane got sick one day. Not all at once, but the illness came to her as a slight discomfort that gradually consumed her until she ended up in a hospital.

But we began in parts. She was studying graphic design in Australia, and when she turned 18 she left Dallas for Australia to pursue a career. For some years she spent there, five to be exact, she made life, developed projects and did very well. Then, when she graduates she decides to come to the United States again, to see her family and decide what her next step would be.

Until then, she was a woman full of talent, joyful, and enterprising like no other.

Being in her city she starts to think about what she should do and opportunities arise in Australia, although it was not what she wanted, it did not fill her need for passion in her life, so she rejects it. Soon, the boyfriend she had at that moment, with whom things were not going well at all, tells her that why not analyze what it is that fills her completely, that makes her happy and that she could do all her life even for free.

For Diane, this is a cold blow because she had never asked herself this before. What it was that moved you that made you think about having the opportunity to achieve something. What her passion was. She had a real talent for many things, she liked graphic design, but it wasn't what she really wanted for her life, she expected more.

She spent several weeks reflecting on what she wanted for her life, she could hardly sleep thinking about what it was that could make her succeed, be a business that she would be in for many years.

Finally, she recognizes that she likes the world of marketing that she could develop a life there, and combined with the design she would earn very well and beyond that, it was something she liked. So she starts working, she sees the strengths and weaknesses in the business and starts to serve several clients, to give them solutions with a company that helps to boost marketing in large corporations.

Soon the clients begin to rain and she must call a friend from Australia, who was her partner for years, he had quite a few projects in the inkwell, but when he hears Diane's proposal he comes, a couple of weeks later they are starting from scratch in the city and giving everything for that business.

So far everything could be fine, but soon Diane's mother gets sick, and during a routine exam, she is found to have early-stage cancer. The operation process to extract it begins and then the chemotherapies, this coincides with the launching of a new product of the company, which generates very high stress. A lot of load, fatigue.

It is there where Diane begins to feel sick, she breaks down, the body feels sore, especially for the legs, which seem to be weaker every day and hurt. She goes to her family doctor, who leaves her in the hospital.

Here she begins a series of medical tests that keep her in bed, checking every part of her body, from her liver to possible pregnancies, cancer, hepatitis, and even yellow fever.

Everything was negative, and every morning they took blood for tests. But even though they saw the physical symptoms, they couldn't make a diagnosis. Her life seemed like a Dr. House chapter, except that after several diagnoses, House did not show up with the origin of the rare disease.

Diane's life was not the best possible right now. They say that illnesses appear because of living conditions; that was what was happening to her. Apparently, she had an illness so severe that she couldn't heal with anything.

Her boyfriend had become insecure and had started to fight over everything, and even when she was in the hospital he didn't miss an opportunity to reproach her for how lonely it felt to have a girlfriend who didn't do that. She was so vulnerable that she actually felt guilty about what was happening to her boyfriend. She asked him to forgive her, even justifying his not visiting her because he claimed that hospitals were the focus of serious illnesses and he did not want to catch them.

She did not say anything, the only thing that went through her mind was that she was to blame for her boyfriend feeling bad, but at the same time deep down there was a spark of anger because the one who should be supporting her in such a hard time was just another executioner.

The relationship was so toxic that they fought several times a day. Even in the moments when she felt the most pain, it was strange that her boyfriend asked her how she was doing. But Diane was a fool, she felt responsible for everything and she put up with it.

In addition to this, her mother was still at home, they didn't see each other because she was undergoing chemotherapy, going to the hospital could be counterproductive and cause her a major condition.

Diane feels deeply alone in this journey because her father was also dedicated to taking care of her mother while she endured the treatments, so all he did was call her, ask her if she wanted him to come, and even though she dreamed of seeing him, she told him it was okay, to continue taking care of her mother.

Her partner and friend also began to push, hoping that one day she would take back the helm of that boat where she had been mounted, so that they could make the very important launch that was frozen thanks to Diane's condition. Everyone seemed to have frozen at that moment. Everything had stopped and Diane's morale began to break down. Being in that hospital, which treated her so well, every day she felt the smells, sounds, and voices coming from every patient. She knew when it was time for the injection because she felt the smell of alcohol nearby, and then a slight groan.

She would hear devices beeping from a routine check-up. His doctor would come every morning and check her legs, and he did so with great care. Even Diane felt a little uncomfortable, but the doctor's face was very professional; he would use a small hammer to hit her in several places and ask her to tell him the degree of pain from one to ten. In the places where it hurt the most it was 7.

But although it seemed that he was being treated as it should, they did not find the evil and she did not fully understand what was happening. Neither did the doctors, although one day she began to understand everything. She realized that the hospital would not heal her. She knew this when the doctor ordered a biopsy, she of course refused and said she was leaving the hospital.

She was not discharged, but she left anyway, although she was affected by having to leave in a wheelchair, a young girl like her, full of vitality, being dragged in a chair. When she arrived home she began to feel a little better and with the passing of the days, the pain began to go away, the reunion with her father, who looked healthier than ever, with her mother who fought like a warrior and looked happy. That warmth of home first helped her get out of bed and walk despite her sore feet, her legs hurt less each day and she started working from her bed.

His partner brought him work and he was checking it out and they were preparing the whole campaign to launch the product. So, eight weeks later a very beautiful Diane was standing at the entrance of the event room, making the launch, was not quite right, but even had recorded content, made writing, and had many ideas for work that would soon be launched.

Months after the launch, when she had already broken up with her toxic boyfriend, she met a young man who was also passionate about marketing, focused, assertive, and soon broke up with her boyfriend. Each one is in their specialty and seems to be doing well. As for her mother, cancer has gone into a very good remission and the prognosis is favorable, it seems that she will be able to sell cancer and the company is not bad at all, they already have several companies in the firm and they continue to arrive, the best thing of all is that Diane is doing what she is most passionate about and each day of work is not a job but a passion where she flies time away and always listens to her satisfied clients.

And about her illness, we never knew what she had because science is not capable of correctly detecting the condition of a person who is sick with stress, and in medical literature, they don't get texts where they say that invisible illnesses exist and that it is not worth the amount of blood they take out, the x-rays or the biopsies, they won't be able to find the evil, because that comes from within, just as Diane had, who upon discovering it, was healed.

Today it is a reference in marketing in the United States and last year it had a revenue of 500 million dollars. They went from two people in the company to manage 236 and the expansions and businesses continue to open every day. Diane's next goal is to get her company listed on the New York Stock Exchange.

She will achieve it, when a woman believes in herself, nothing stops her.

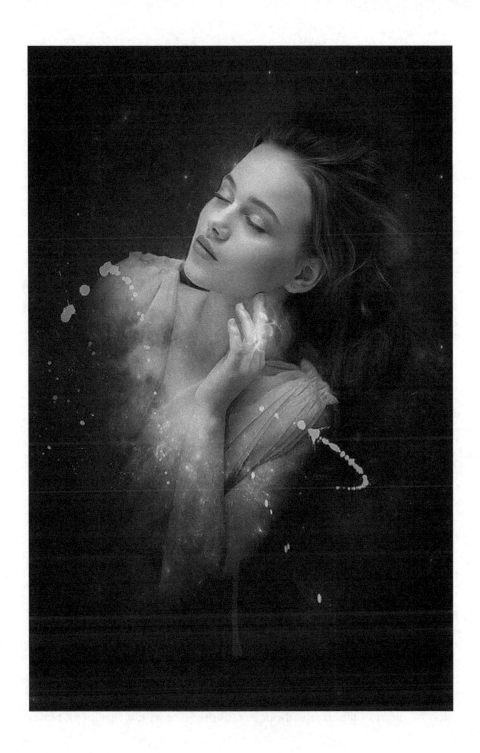

The Intermittence of Love

There are love stories that are made by the gods themselves, who pull the strings so that the relationships are those special ones that inspire the most beautiful verses and the most romantic stories.

The story that we are going to narrate next has as its main character Abril, who met a boy of her same age, she was older than him for some months, but he has the advantage of being more mature in many things, he has had a difficult life that has forced him to see life in a different way than many people of his age.

April, from the first moment that she connected with him, always sought to stand out, to give him the impression that she was interested in him, she talked to him, she was interested in his life and little by little she showed him the alarm that yes, she was available to be seduced to show that she was open to a relationship.

The first subtle signs didn't have much effect, but little by little he became aware of her interest and Brian realized that he liked her too. That's when the flirting started and he was surprised that he liked April so much and that she reciprocated like no other.

She would open up to show her interest in him, you could see it when they were talking and talking about sex, he would ask what he liked and she would say some things that she liked and he would let it be known that he did not like to talk about sex, but that he would surely not regret it.

Brian was a suspicious man, many people had failed him, and so for a woman to come and talk to him so openly about sex and that everything he saw seemed perfect, he was overwhelmed, where did such a perfect woman come from, the truth could not be like that. He did not deserve it, or so he thought.

Although men have the particularity of feeling the distrust, but not lose the opportunity to go to bed with the woman and this made it clear one day when he said:

—Let's meet up and go to a hotel, see what happens, let whatever fate desires happen.

So, they planned to meet and Brian took her to dinner, then he took her to a cozy, romantic hotel with a bed full of rose petals and candles, a service that was paid for and that he put there to celebrate with her.

The atmosphere was perfect for the two of them to make love with passion, both of them walking around and getting to know each other's curves, the perfections and imperfections, smelling each other, tasting each other, and getting to know each other's sounds in the games of love. As if they were a pair of old souls, the bodies met again and enjoyed as in no moment the two had done. This made her immensely happy, she felt very much loved by him, and wanted to be the beloved of this man who did not lose any centimeter to go through her.

Brian liked it, very much, because the pleasure was immense, but he knew deep down that they were not ero sex, there was also within them a taste that increased and they liked it, that no matter how expert you can be in sex there is always a connection that cannot be explained, that is not love yet, but that connects and makes those souls become one.

That's how the two of them were and soon they fell in love, although as the relationship grew and they fell more in love, Brian began to feel a lot of anxiety, at first he didn't know, but he woke up even at night with that fear stuck in his chest, he slept without understanding for sure what was happening to him, but soon, he began to be dazzled by what was happening to him, was first like a spark, like a minimal flame that told him that something was happening inside, that it could be that his base, the comfort zone that he had established and where he felt safe, was beginning to crack and he was coming to an abyss from which it might be difficult to get out, that he could stay forever in that hole, that he could return to that time where he had so many vulnerabilities.

One morning after having stayed up for several hours, he deduced that he was afraid to feel so comfortable with her. With his girlfriend, with April, having such a divine time made him feel bad, because the alarm that this woman was too perfect was going off.

That's why the first time he makes the mistake is when he goes and impulsively blocks her from the cell phone and social networks.

Poor April did not know what to do because one night they talked like the most in love in the world and the next day the man had vanished, when he went to say good morning, the profile photo of the WhatsApp was in a gray face and on social networks did not appear, called him and sounded a beep, characteristic that had been blocked, in short, the man vanished. April was not a woman to stay tied, so she went immediately to take her brother's cell phone and called him, this number was not in

Brian's possession, so he answered.

The man didn't know what to answer, he babbled and Abril demanded to see him right away in person and told him that she was going out to meet him, after a while, he came home.

When they were already in person he explained to her that the best thing was to leave this until here, but he didn't give her any reason and Abril wasn't going to be left with a simple breakup, where she didn't say anything, she wanted him to make it very clear what was happening to him. And in the end, after asking many questions, he ended up showing his fear and telling her that he felt insecure, that she was a very perfect woman to be real, that he couldn't speak so well, be so loving, so good a lover, she came from many gestures and seemed to be unconditional "such a perfect woman cannot exist".

She promised him that she would love him for a long time, that he was the love of her life, that nothing would end, that they were eternal, that she would not leave that relationship, and that she would not let it end, because she knew what he felt and he knew what she felt that if they could even give themselves to love right now, live, have children, whatever he wanted, because Brian was the love of her life, because they wouldn't separate for anything in the world, that's how he made it clear to them, and they started making love right there, making up, and he felt safe and a fool because he had thought that way.

The social networks were restored, the number was unblocked and they started the love relationship again. All happy, in a great springtime they celebrated by going out to make love, to enjoy, to eat, to go to many places.

Love was back to normal, but Brian put it all together again, thinking about why she had been so loving in the reconciliation, then said she was insane, maybe she was a crazy person who had an obsession, like Norman Bates, the psychopath in Psycho, who would one day kill him and talk to him like his mother, while renting a room in a road hotel.

That's what he thought, full of fear, full of anguish, so the more loving she was to him, again he would behave as if he had fears, as if she were a traitor.

Then another day he didn't block her, but he was very harsh with her, he told her that they were breaking up, that no, that the explanations were too much, that the relationship was going to hell, and that goodbye. So, without anesthesia, with a lot of pain for her, she broke down, cried a lot, felt miserable because her man was leaving her and Brian took it upon himself to be such a scoundrel, to hurt her in such a brutal way that her ego was so bruised that they left each other. He did not block her from the networks, so they checked social networks, looked at photos, she sometimes left him a "like" to show that there was love. It was a very big feeling, they finally ended up talking, they ended up together.

Three years went by, several times he left her, they spent a couple of months apart, she cried a lot, and she was torn. With a lot of pain. At night, before going to sleep, he would hug her, kiss her, and feel that she was very far away. He was very much in love, but he wasn't able to do it. He felt the love, he felt the desire, but there was always the latent fear.

One day, April tired of that insecurity told him to go to hell, so, with that scatological word, when he showed that everything was going to end because he felt that there were failures, she threw him out, that now if they finished. He felt very sad, because he loved his beloved deeply and hoped, as was his custom, that she would beg him. But he did not admit it, he told her that he agreed, that they were ending.

The love was over forever, she thought. That weekend, she went out and accepted that person who showed her desire, they saw each other and in the midst of spite April allowed him to kiss her, but the mouth of that man did not know her love, the smell was not the same, the texture of his skin, nothing, she felt disgusted, as if she were a prostitute who kissed the client on duty, then separated from that man and left.

She was anchored to that sickly relationship of an insecure man who couldn't put on his pants, who couldn't show that there was real love, who couldn't accept being loved, an insecure man who had always been cheated on, so when someone sincere showed up he wasn't able to enjoy himself, a little man, a silly scoundrel.

The Habit

Holly and Bolton have been married for several years. How does a couple get used to doing the same thing over and over again without wanting to kill each other?

They met one night in a bar, they were the roll of a Friday, two unknown people, they liked each other, they understood each other in bed and the next day they each went on with their lives. They said that they had nothing more to say to each other, that they had to get on with their lives and that this was just a one-night stand, they both agreed and both forgot

About a month later they met again in a bar, they talked and felt a different vibration, the two had desires for each other, and they found themselves in bed again, wishing each other, wanting to have sex, at dawn they said goodbye again forever, saying that it had been an exception to the rule

The point is that they kept meeting, they kept seeing each other and they liked each other more and more and the sexual encounters were more intense.

Soon they got into the habit of having these encounters, even though they said they lived somewhat sporadically, the encounter took place in a bar, they ended up in the same hotel, and repeated the same movements in bed, they even got to a point of having the same room, they already knew the scars on the walls and the sounds in the mattress, the trick of the key when opening and the exact point to make it warm as they liked, they knew the steps that separated the door of the room from the ice machine and the time when the maid spent the next day collecting the dirt and cleaning rooms.

They made a habit of doing the same thing and repeated it. One day, they began to get tired of these supposedly accidental encounters, and scheduled a date outside the party environment, invited her to dinner. They went to a fish place, where they ate some sea paella that they both liked with a white wine recommended by the chef, they got to know each other better, she was aspiring to be an actress, he was composing songs and selling them to different musicians, her wish was that one of those lyrics would be bought by some famous singer.

There was romance in the air, they already knew each other's skins and knew they understood each other well, although until then they were a bit drunk. That night, after dinner, they went to a better hotel, one that did not have the walls so thin as to filter the sound from the neighboring rooms.

With a bed that had no sound and a TV that had more than porn channels. For the first time, they made love with romance, they carefully walked around giving each other pleasure, fell asleep hugging like an old married couple, kissed at dawn, and made love in the shower.

They ordered breakfast from the room and continued the encounter for many more hours, walking unhurriedly, discovering each other, and giving way to what would be a nascent relationship. Soon they were formal boyfriends, and the meetings were not so common in a hotel, but began to go to galleries, concerts, he received her in the failed auditions that were all, never called, some were deceptive offers to work as a prostitute and encouraged her when she decided to start working in a cafe.

On Mondays, they did not see each other because he went to an event, on Tuesdays they met after seven o'clock when she left work, on Wednesdays it was repeated, on Thursdays they did not see each other because it was the night where she met with other failed actors, on Fridays they met and spent the weekend at his house, eating pizza, reheated food and watching series on shift. Two years passed in this cycle, repeating the ritual without changes except for extraordinary exceptions.

After a fight, on her part, because she was tired of the same thing, he solved everything with an engagement ring, which was kept for a year and a half by more than one engaged couple to be able to step up to the altar.

Another fight put a date on it, now, the happy couple was on the same roof, with the same bills and the commitments. She wanted children, but he was not prepared, two years went by and many fights to make them take the step and start making love in every corner to be able to get pregnant.

Six months later, she was given the miracle, she had a delay, they bought a pregnancy test and it was positive, nine months later a little boy was born who changed the dynamics of the home, and the custom began to fall apart, they did not do so much the same things, but tried new experiences.

As the child grew, they tried other things, but when the little one reached seven years of age everything returned to the routine, the man came home from work and started watching television, he did not share with the little one, the latter asked him to play, to do new things, but he did not attend to him, his mother did not attend to him either, she was on her cell phone, complaining about her husband who did not attend to the child or to her.

They say you become the person you surround yourself with, Holly was, a female version of her husband, now she was living in the same cycle of routines, of procrastinating and doing the same thing over and over again. The boy reached adolescence, built his world, and walked with his friends, except to get to sleep, the young man was never at home.

Married, immersed in routine, everything seemed normal to him, they lived at their own pace, doing their own things, each one living in the routines. They had already established them, she did the chores, he put the food on, watched TV and talked a little about work, he had given up music, he was frustrated like Holly who was never an actress.

Without fail, every Saturday night, he would caress her, kiss her and repeat the same route, putting his hand through some folds, running his tongue through others, opening with his fingers, entering, giving himself the same amount of movements, she would have a mechanical orgasm or sometimes she would fake it and he would finish soon after, she would wash and he would wipe himself with paper.

They would watch TV as if nothing had happened, half an hour later he would fall asleep and she would change and put on some channel that she liked, when she was sleepy she would fall asleep and so on until Sunday, when he would wake up after ten o'clock, she had already made breakfast, had lunch on the way and the house was clean.

She would read the newspaper, while she was having breakfast, the time would be tied up with lunch, when she ate, they would go to bed to watch some series together, take naps, drink coffee and the routine of the week would start on Monday, until Friday again.

It was a routine of years that although it seemed that neither of them cared, it was already boring, he did not care about her, if they asked him he would realize that he did not care much, he did not love her, if she was missing the only thing he would miss would be the habit of seeing her there.

She loved him, but since she had a lot of love, she was immensely bored by the man, thinking about him made her want to yawn, she knew what he was going to say, she could almost imitate him because every sentence he said on every day of the week she knew by heart, sometimes she was ahead of what he was going to ask because she already knew he would ask.

Whoever has never been married could say that this marriage was doomed to failure, but no, it was the typical American marriage and from many parts of the world, eternal couples who were stuck in their own comfort zones and even though they were extremely boring they felt at ease.

Old age caught up with them and with it the routines, with age people acquire strange customs, old manias, they called it. She got used to being with the man with his accidental farts, he had gotten used to a woman who gave hostile answers, the product of the age that allowed him not to shut up at all.

The two would die together, one would die first than the other, their son would come every now and then to visit them, bringing them food, because they no longer worked, now with them at home all the time, the habits were more intense, the customs were more accentuated. He watched TV all day, took a dog they had out for a walk, fed the pigeons in a park, and, like an old cat, slept all afternoon.

Arranging socks, arranging clothes, and looking for what to do, the habit of being active prevented her from living the lazy life her husband had. As for the two of them, they could spend the whole day close by, next to each other, and not talk, not because they were angry at all, but because they were used to their presence.

And after so many years of marriage, there is not much to say to each other, and when they do not do anything transcendental, they do not have much to say to each other, except that a dove shat the dog, or that the dog beat the buttock of a child, or she hurt her thumb with a needle, or that the grinder locked again.

Habits are the best glue for eternal love.

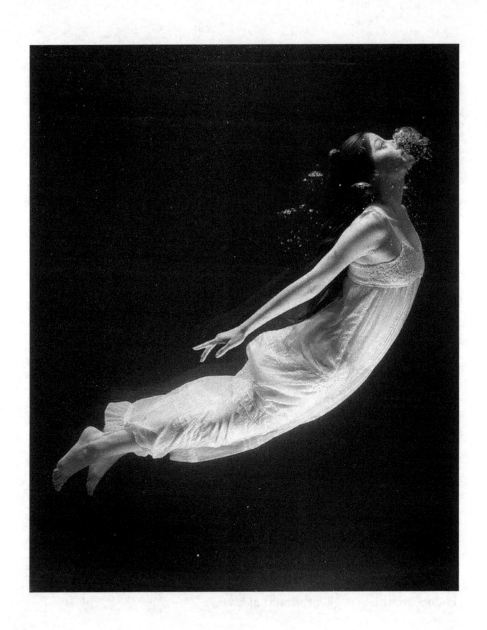

The Bed

Daryl was married, he had a wife with whom he had lived for fifteen years, an ordinary marriage that doesn't deserve many lines, because you would yawn from boredom. The relationship already had so many cracks that he had chosen to have one of those lovers who behaves like girlfriends and does everything that regular women don't. In exchange, he gave her what she needed, money for her expenses, the rent for the cell phone, the house and to buy her cleaning supplies.

His lover was a 19-year-old white girl with pink lips, thin and contoured legs, a beautiful body with round breasts and small nipples, who would hump when she made love and do what no one else had done to her that purred like no other that had him in love lusting after that woman with intensity.

Every Wednesday, he would tell his mother that he would go bowling and go to the small apartment he had with his lover and they would make love, eat, talk and behave like a couple of boyfriends. Daryl was getting younger with Crystal, looking forward to that day every week.

The relationship could have continued without the setbacks, if something hadn't started happening in his life. On one visit while he was in bed with her, he felt warmer than usual, even though he had just gone to bed. Normally, when you first lie down in bed, you feel the cloth cold, at room temperature, but soon, the body heat makes it warm. When a person lies down on a bed that has just been vacated, it feels warm, the residual heat of the body. That's what he felt that first time.

He didn't say anything, at that moment he had Crystal undressing and devouring him with kisses, but days later, already calm, he began to think about Crystal's bed, to make conjectures about what could be happening, tying up loose ends, thinking about if under the bed could have been a naked man listening to what she was saying in the midst of the passion she considered her girlfriend. For his own sanity, he preferred to think that everything had been the object of his insecurity.

Many nights, when his wife was sleeping and he heard her soft snoring, and he took the opportunity to use his cell phone, but also to write to Crystal, he usually answered her immediately and they talked for a long time, what every lover says, words of love, hot conversations, some pictures of her, to put it, telling her he wanted it. There were days when she would write him hot messages, with pictures, make up a whole hot story and then, when she had it melted, ask him for something. She was no saint, she knew how to get anything from her man.

The following Wednesday, he went to see her, he had in his unconscious the idea of the bed, from the living room while they were talking he saw it out of the corner of his eye, he even detailed it underneath, it was empty, they talked, kissed, had dinner and went to bed, when she sat down she felt him warm, I could say even warmer than the previous week. He said nothing, but felt uncomfortable the whole encounter because he could not enjoy his beloved. Many theories were going through his head about what could be the reason for that bed to be warm.

The question became more critical, because as the weeks went by the bed became hotter and hotter, to the point that one night he found it so hot that it was difficult to get into it.

—What's wrong, love? Come to bed, this kitten is waiting for you.

The woman would wiggle around half-naked and ask him to get into bed. The man did not want to give in, the temptation was great, but he was eager to know what was happening.

—This bed is on fire.

—Of course, if I'm in it, it's on fire, waiting for you.

—No, it's not that, it's literally hot.

—I don't understand you.

—The bed, touch it, it's hot.

Crystal touched, raised her shoulders as if to imply that she was normal.

—Every week I sell I feel the bed getting hotter, right now it's about to burn, I don't know how you're standing on it.

—Love, have you gone crazy? Every week I wait anxiously for you and now that I'm here, all for you, you go crazy.

She said that and opened her legs, showing her panty and inviting him to come, Daryl took her, lifted her and placed her on the couch in the living room, they made love there, she felt excited because they were trying new things, doing it in other places, he forgot for a while that he had left the bed because it was burning without knowing for what reason. When they finished, they went to take a bath, when they went out, without her noticing, she touched the bed and it was cold, it was as if no one had been in it all day.

He didn't understand what was going on, but this put him in a bad mood, because he knew that something was hiding behind this situation, the woman could be hiding something or he was going crazy.

That week he was in a bad mood, thinking the worst, when she didn't immediately respond to his messages he imagined the worst that Crystal was with another man in bed, that he had his turn on Wednesdays and everyone had their turn to be with her. The bad mood was unbearable, he fought with his wife a couple of times, all because of him, who responded badly to the woman's comments.

At work, he was in a bad mood, his subordinates couldn't stand him, they were afraid to even talk to him. When he arrived on Wednesday, he arrived a little earlier at her house, but he did not get out of the car, but stayed there watching, after a while, he realized that the woman was not hiding anything, he even wrote her a message that where he was then he got out, entered the house and shared with her, the bed was warm again, not burning like the previous week, but it seemed to have been occupied. They made love, ordered pizza, and that night, for the first time in their lives, he slept with her, it wasn't planned, they were hugging, talking, one was silent, then the other and they fell asleep.

The next day, at six o'clock in the morning, he went home quickly, his wife would surely be furious, what would be his surprise when he arrived, she greeted him as if nothing had happened and went to sleep for a while, then she bathed, went to work and his wife did not even bother to ask him where he had spent the night.

The suspicions with Crystal did not end, one night, not Wednesday, he went to her house, parked half a block away, and dedicated himself to observe, attentive to see if anything happened, the house was quiet, nobody went out, nobody entered. The next day he did the same thing, only this time he got off and went over to the house, tried to listen, looked behind the curtain, saw her pass by, into the kitchen, she looked lonely. Even the day he saw her pass by with her cell phone in her hand, he jumped up and down, because at the moment he wrote to her, the woman seemed to be open only to him.

Other nights he went to visit her, they shared and continued their eternal romance with a beautiful spring. Daryl decided one day to do something risky, he called her and told her to get ready, that he would go get her, it was a Friday, he was already waiting for her outside the house, but she didn't say anything, he had her tested. The woman left on time, beautiful as ever, they went to dinner and returned, that night again he stayed with her at home, the next morning, this time without worrying about the woman's reaction, he arrived at mid-morning, it was Saturday, so he settled in his bed and slept all day. His wife didn't even claim him.

The encounters continued and Crystal's bed was still warm, but it hadn't gotten as hot as it had weeks before. Although he watched her, he never saw another man in her house and everything she said seemed to be real, he didn't pretend to hide anything and the lover's relationship that now moved on to something more formal, seemed not to displease him, on the contrary, he seemed at ease.

One day, the bed simply stopped being warm, it was as if this whole episode had never happened, by chance it started to be normal when he fell more in love with Crystal and wanted to live with her, to share his life with that young woman. He took the step, he didn't care, he was even determined to send his wife to hell. He was considering asking her for a divorce, it would be the best thing to do to move to Crystal's house for good.

The day he proposed it to his lover, she was thrilled, she liked the idea of having him there every day, not sleeping alone every night. She had also not been indifferent to the attachment they had had in recent times, so she gladly accepted.

Daryl stayed at her house, the next day he arrived home, ready to talk to his wife, she didn't ask him where he was, he took a bath, changed and went out to look for his wife, he couldn't find her, he missed her going out, he went into the bedroom, checked the closet and saw that she had put on the dress she used for special dates, one he had given her years ago, it was a signature dress and it looked beautiful.

She missed it, but she didn't give it much thought, she went to bed, as soon as she sat down on it, she had to get up, it was burning, like embers, she put her hand twenty centimeters closer and felt the steam in her palm.

Sometimes the games are mutual.

The Infinite Thread of Drinks

After leaving work he walked to the street where he usually walked. He knew every inch of that place, although he hadn't stepped on it for fifteen years. There he stayed, looking at his premises, seeing that time had not passed through them, although the faces he saw were new, deciding whether to go home or stay there, he had needed to come to this street for quite some time.

He walked to the place he had always visited, he knew it well, he stopped at the door and detailed it, there are countless times he left there totally drunk, he sighed, he knew he had no choice, so he went in. The interior of the place was also identical to how he remembered it, the usual bad-smelling tables, the people sitting there drinking and thinking about their things, some happy playing dominoes, others talking at full speed and at the back the bar, where their hunched backs drank slowly. He went and took the chair that was available, sat down, and looked at the man who was attending, it took him several seconds to recognize him, he was the same barman as always, grayer, with more belly and wrinkles.

The man looked at him, contemplated for a while that face that was familiar to him, but he also had more wrinkles and weight.

—Collins? —he asked. —The same, and as handsome as ever.

—I thought I'd never see you again.

—You see. Give me the usual.

The man, as if he had just seen him the day before, walked over, took the bottle of white rum, and poured the first drink of the night into his glass.

In another life, Collins never left this place. Every night when he finished work, he would come to the bar and his dinner would be rum until he felt his head spinning, walked home, went to bed, and stood up when the alarm clock was beating his head. He could have been like that all his life, with a permanent hangover and poor nutrition, if it weren't for the fact that one day he met the woman who is now his wife, the woman he loves most in the world. They fell in love, had three children, and today they are happy together.

Although the happiness is never complete, although Collins adores his wife, takes care of her and even at the time he agreed with her and promised never to drink in this way again, today he is here, pouring rum again and with a pain in his heart. As he drinks the rum he feels guilt, he knows that he is disappointing his wife, that he is failing her. She would feel sad if she saw him drinking.

At the same time he feels anger, because his wife is the one who caused him to be there at this moment, Collins is hurt, he has been in a bad mood for days, he is grumpier than usual and those who know Collins know that the man is the noblest thing in the world, kind, respectful, always talking in a slow tone, without saying bad words and without attacking, but right now he is full of anger, now he cares very little about everything and that is why he asks for another drink from his favorite barman.

Think about how difficult it is for a man to be the head of the family, to always have a good attitude knowing that you have debts, that the mortgage is coming, that the child needs shoes, that the wife wants that dress, that two months ago you don't go to the park or the mall or to that attraction that came to town, these are so many things and as a father you want to fulfill them all like that, so don't even say thank you.

Collins has sought to comply and many nights he goes to bed proud of himself, of having complied like a good father, of having given his children what they needed and of smiling at feeling part of these achievements, that's what he thinks, that's what he feels.

What is the reason that brings Collins to this bar after fifteen years? What happens every time he comes home, the being the good guy in the family, but the woman puts him in the place as the villain, and tells him that the boy did such a mischief, that she was waiting for him to scold him or that the other one broke the glass while playing with the ball.

Then, Collins, who came with the tiredness weighing on his soul, who was eager to get home, kiss his wife and stroke the children's hair to ask her how the day was going, has to put on his villain's face and scold the children for mischief that he doesn't even care about, He does it because that is what husbands have to do, to support each other, if he takes his wife's complaint as something frugal, then she will be angry for several days, will tell him that she is alone for everything and the man will feel sad. He regrets so much that after a day of work he has to come to deal with things in the home that are his responsibility, he wonders what his wife's desire is to make him the villain, he is not the villain, he is the man who loves his children, the one who wants to play, once he came with the desire to play ball with the little one, to see how he was standing out, to take a few shots and to talk.

He was born as a father to do that and when his wife arrived, she told him that the little one had done a mischief and there was his prince, looking at him with a guilty face and Collins took out of where he did not have a rage to claim that mischief, he sent him to his room and was left with a heavy heart seeing his little one goes into his room, he had been left with the desire to play with him, with the desire to make him feel that he loved him, his wife did not even notice, she just wanted to get revenge and she got it.

That's why he drinks, because he doesn't want to go to that house where his wife waits for him with more complaints, claims, showing what he did or didn't do with a certain child, denying that such a child needs two straps, that the other one has to be punished, and he's there drinking because for days he has wanted to stay by the woman's side and yell at her to fuck off, that he's not a villain, that he doesn't have to make her beat the children for something she doesn't even care about. He wants to say it, but he is so angry that he prefers to control himself, he knows that if he opens his mouth he will scream, he will say bad words, he will hurt.

When he feels that the liquor is filling his head, he gets up, says goodbye to his lifelong bartender, and tells him that someday they will meet again. He leaves feeling the liquor in his head, today he didn't drink much, but so many years without stepping on this place besides the age he was, it was enough to make his mind foggy and get drunk faster than before.

A short time later he put the key in the door of his house, opened it, inside there was his wife, who was shouting something to one of the rooms, when she saw him, her greeting was:

—When he saw it, his greeting was: Thank goodness you've arrived, where were you? You have to scold that son of yours, he just gave me a bad face because I asked him to eat everything. Go and tell him something because he obeys you

—Why don't you make yourself obey then?

—How do you say?

—That I don't have to be the villain of the film that you can be.

—Do you think I don't spend all day putting them on the track, but they don't listen, they don't obey, only you.

—Make yourself respected.

—Do you smell liquor? —said his wife, making a sad face.

—Yes, I smell liquor, so what?

—You promised never to drink again.

—I'm fed up.

—Sick of what?

—Of coming to this house every day and having to put up with you making me mistreat the children, do you think I don't want to hug them? I want to play with them, not punish them, the problems they have had can be solved by you, you don't have to get me into that mess, if I come exhausted from work, with so many things on my mind, I don't have to add to that having to fight with my little ones, I just want to play.

—What are you talking about?

—I'm not going to scold my children anymore, not for things they haven't done to me.

That night Collins slept on the furniture, it was to be expected that his wife did not understand, although she lasted some days annoyed, at the worst she understood that she did not count on her husband to make them feel the authority and Collins did not return to the bar, every night he came home to play with his children and although the woman threw hints, he ignored them and enjoyed his little ones because he knew that in a sigh they would be gone, they would be with their own lives and he would have missed an important stage of their lives because of senseless fights invented by his wife.

Sometimes the parents are put as the villains to be able to raise the children and not always the parents want to be them, what more they wish in many occasions is to be able to arrive home to embrace their children and to rest for some hours of the hustle and bustle of the day.